FIND YOUR ANIMAL SIDE

Coloring Book & Yoga Guide

Veronica McDaniel
& Sarah Bristow

Printed by CreateSpace, an Amazon.com Company

DEDICATION PAGE

We dedicate this book to our supportive
husbands, Mark McDaniel and Austin Bristow.

TABLE OF CONTENTS

1 Preface

2 Introduction

3-4 Butterfly

5-6 Camel

7-8 Cat

9-10 Cobra

11-12 Cow

13-14 Crow

15-16 Dolphin

17-18 Downward Dog

19-20 Eagle

21-22 Firefly

23-24 Fish

25-26 Flamingo

27-28 Frog

29-30 Horse

31-32 Lion's Breath

33-34 Locust

35-36 Pigeon

37-38 Rabbit

39-40 Shark

41-42 Tortoise

43-47 Glossary

47-48 Notes Page

49-50 Design Your Own Sequence

PREFACE

VERONICA:

Ever since Veronica was a kid she loved drawing ink and colored pencil drawings. She considered pursuing an Art career and ultimately it has remained a hobby. Recently, Veronica was inspired to create original artwork which serves as a guide to something that people can use independently and that supports a healthy, purposeful lifestyle. As a Secondary School Physical Education teacher, staying fit is an innate passion. On an early morning run she was inspired to merge her interest in drawing and fitness with her running buddy Sarah's growing passion of teaching kids yoga and mindfulness. She embarked on drawing for this book and spent a few months drawing each evening and loving every minute of it. Veronica set out to create something that would entice kids to adults alike. She envisions this book for people of all ages to enjoy on their leisure time in order to wind down and appreciate the little things each day has to offer.

SARAH:

Health and wellness have always been a priority for Sarah. You can often find her running, cycling, hiking, and spending time with her husband and two young children. By day she is a passionate educator and mentor, and she spends evenings with her family playing outside and preparing healthy meals. With ten years of elementary school teaching experience, Sarah seeks to creatively integrate health into the classroom. From teaching mindful moments within the school community to making cold pressed juices with ingredients from the school garden, Sarah is an advocate for nourishing the body and mind. Yoga and mindfulness are paramount to her own daily wellness plan and she is dedicated to sharing this with others. The weekend classes and workshops Sarah teaches typically begin by coloring a mandala as a way of tuning. Veronica's first drawing of a deeply rooted tree (seen on the back cover) became the foundation for Sarah's practice, Growing Grounded. Since then, Sarah and Veronica have shared ideas about yoga and art which ultimately led to collaboration on this project. (www.growinggrounded.org)

ACKNOWLEDGEMENTS:

Artists Dora McDaniel and Olga Plaut; editor Robert Shaw-Smith; scanner John McCusker; consultant Nicole O'Brien; graphic designer Ana de Olano; critics Lana, Mateo; and the Bartlett family.

INTRODUCTION

Life gets busy! This book was created to help you find stillness in your day by connecting with your creative side. We hope to inspire budding artists and yogis of all ages. As you explore the different drawings and poses, we encourage you to put pencil to paper and step onto your mat to try something new. You just may surprise yourself.

Feel free to move through the poses in this book in any order and add other poses as you see fit. We encourage you to create your own sequences and listen to your body as you work. The descriptions offer introductory instruction with options to advance your practice. Please reference the Glossary images for visuals of the poses, visit the Notes page to write down your own thoughts, and use the Sequence pages to create the sequences that flow best for you.

CAUTION: If you are pregnant please consult a physician before practicing. For those with any sort of medical condition please consult a medical practitioner and a yoga teacher to avoid any dangers or difficulties that may arise.

BUTTE

R T L Y
(BADDHA KONASANA)

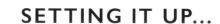

ABOUT THE STRETCH...

Stimulates abdominal organs, ovaries and prostate gland, bladder, and kidneys. Also stimulates the heart and improves general circulation. Stretches the inner thighs, groins, and knees. Helps relieve mild depression, anxiety, fatigue, and symptoms of menopause. Traditional texts claim that Baddha Konasana gets rid of disease and fatigue.

SETTING IT UP...

From a seated position, bring your heels in toward your pelvis, letting your knees fall open. Press the soles of your feet together.

Grasp the big toe of each foot with the first and second finger and thumb. Keep the outer edges of the feet firmly on the floor (modification is to hold onto the shins.)

Lengthen up through the crown of your head.

Poses to precede this pose are Supta Padangusthasana *(reclining hand to big toe pose)*, Hero Pose, and Tree Pose. Often followed by Seated Twists and forward bends.

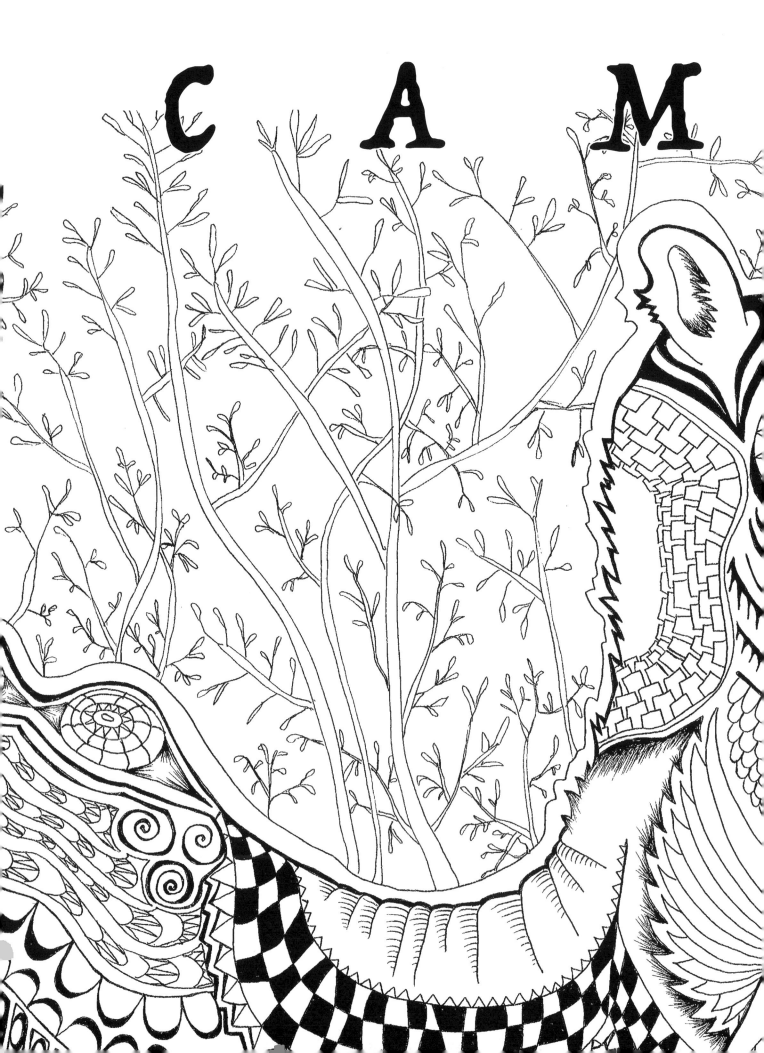

E L

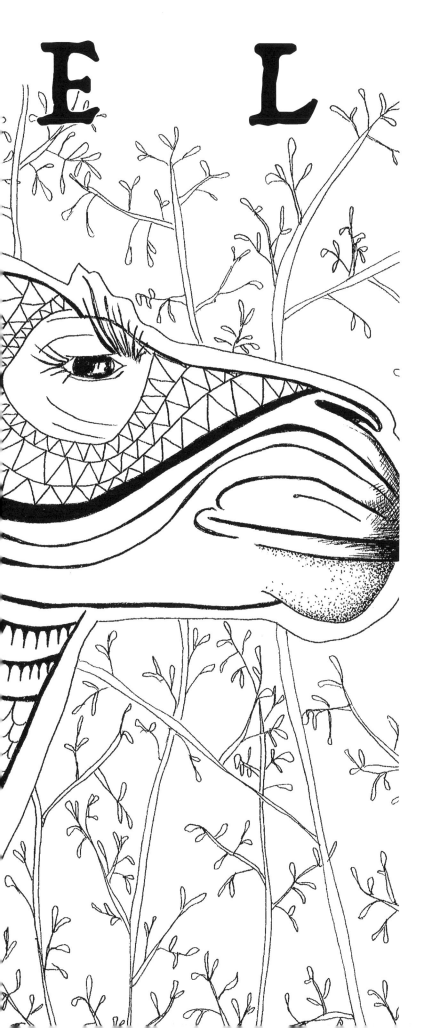

(USTRASANA)

ABOUT THE STRETCH...

Stretches the entire front of the body, from the ankles up to the throat. Strengthens back muscles and improves posture. Stimulates the organs of the abdomen and neck, improving digestion and elimination. Opens the chest, improving respiration.

SETTING IT UP...

Kneel on the floor with your knees hip width and thighs perpendicular to the floor. Press your shins and the tops of your feet firmly into floor.

Rest your hands on the back of your pelvis, bases of the palms on the tops of the buttocks with fingers pointing down. Press your front thighs back, countering the forward action of your tail pulling downward.

Inhale and lift your heart by pressing the shoulder blades back. Lean back against the tail bone and shoulder blades.

Deepen? Continue tilting back and gently twist to one side to reach the same side foot. Then come back to neutral and touch the second hand to its foot.

Sit back into Hero Pose and prepare for Bridge or Full Wheel.

6

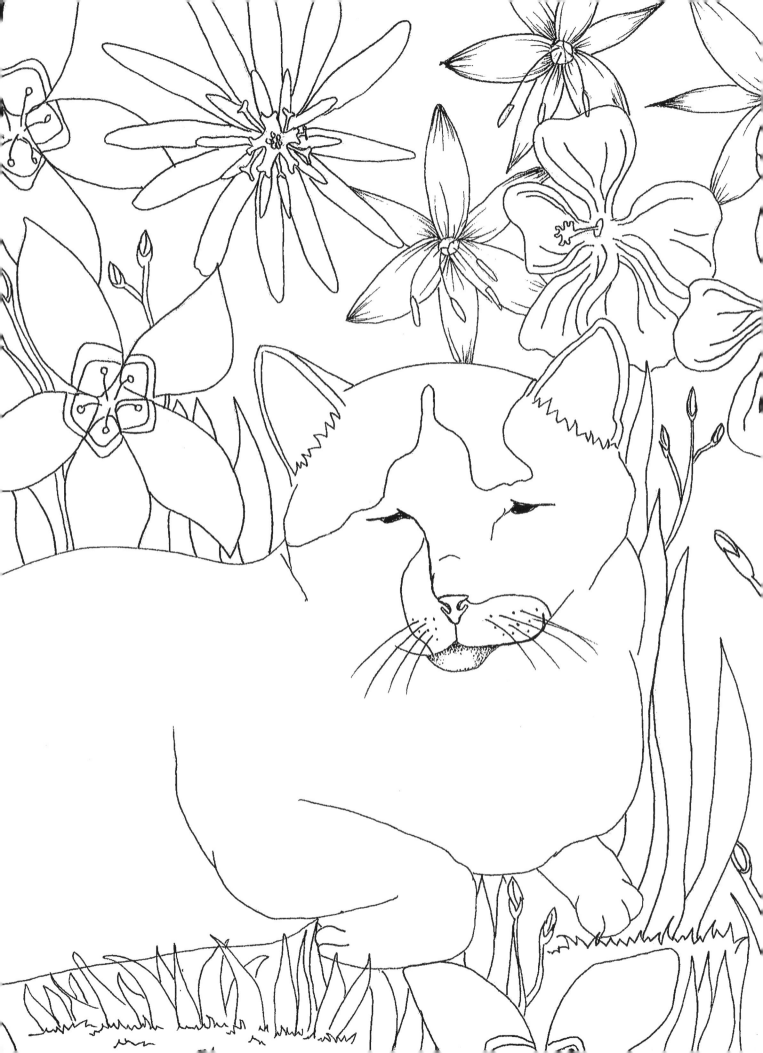

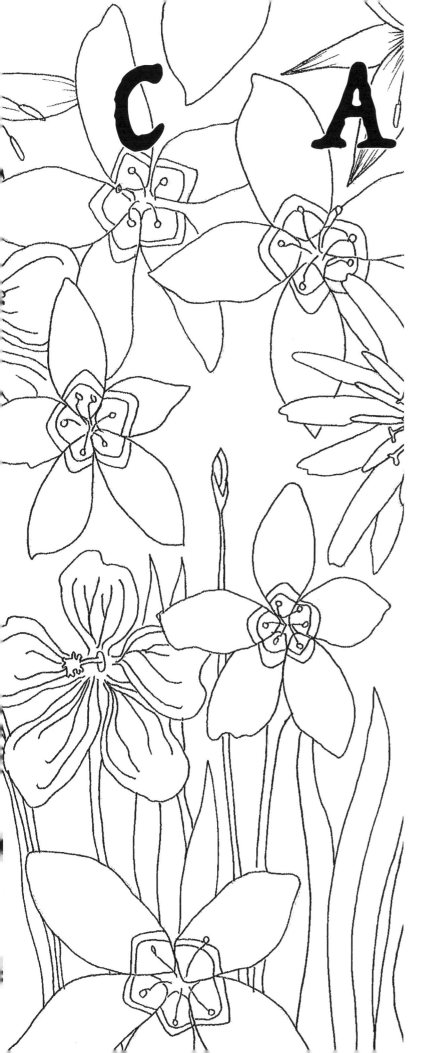

C A T

(MARJARI)

ABOUT THE STRETCH...

Strengthens and stretches the spine and neck while stretching the hips, abdomen and back. Massages and stimulates organs in the belly such as the kidneys and adrenal glands. Also known to increase coordination.

SETTING IT UP...

From your hands and knees (Tabletop Position) align your hips with your knees to maintain a neutral spine. Firmly press your palms into the ground beneath your shoulders.

Breathe in, and as you exhale, lower your head, tuck your hips down and curve your spine inward and upward. Think of "rounding your back."

Cat and Cow pair well together as part of a gentle Vinyasa flow (series of movements between poses.) Add Twisted Puppy for an additional stretch.

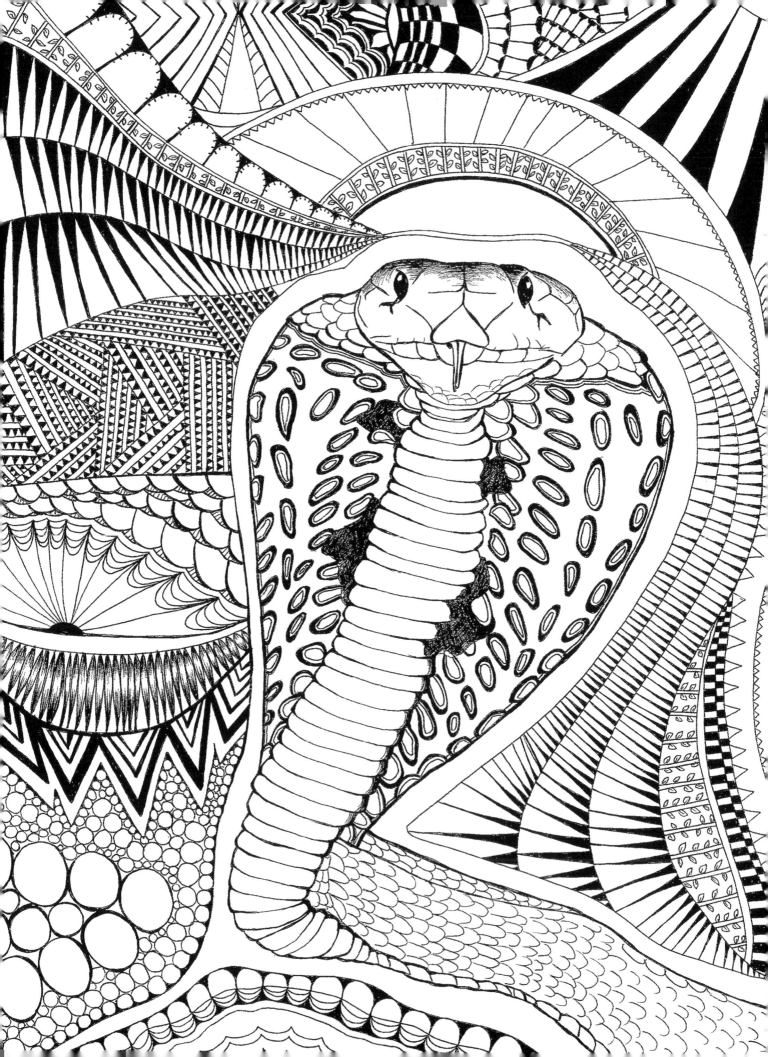

COBRA
(BHUJANGASANA)

ABOUT THE STRETCH...
Relieves discomfort in the back, neck and abdominal muscles. Additionally, it can alleviate stress, anxiety, and depression.

SETTING IT UP...
Laying on your stomach, place the tops of your feet close together and flat on the ground.

Plant your hands just outside your shoulders, fingers spread wide, and hug your elbows into your ribs.

Inhale and lift your chest up off the ground, opening across your chest. Exhale and lower down slowly.

Cobra is part of the Sun Salutation flow (warm up sequence to prepare for practice.) Lower down through Chaturanga (a yoga push-up), lift into Cobra Pose, and breathe before tucking your toes inward and returning to Downward Facing Dog.

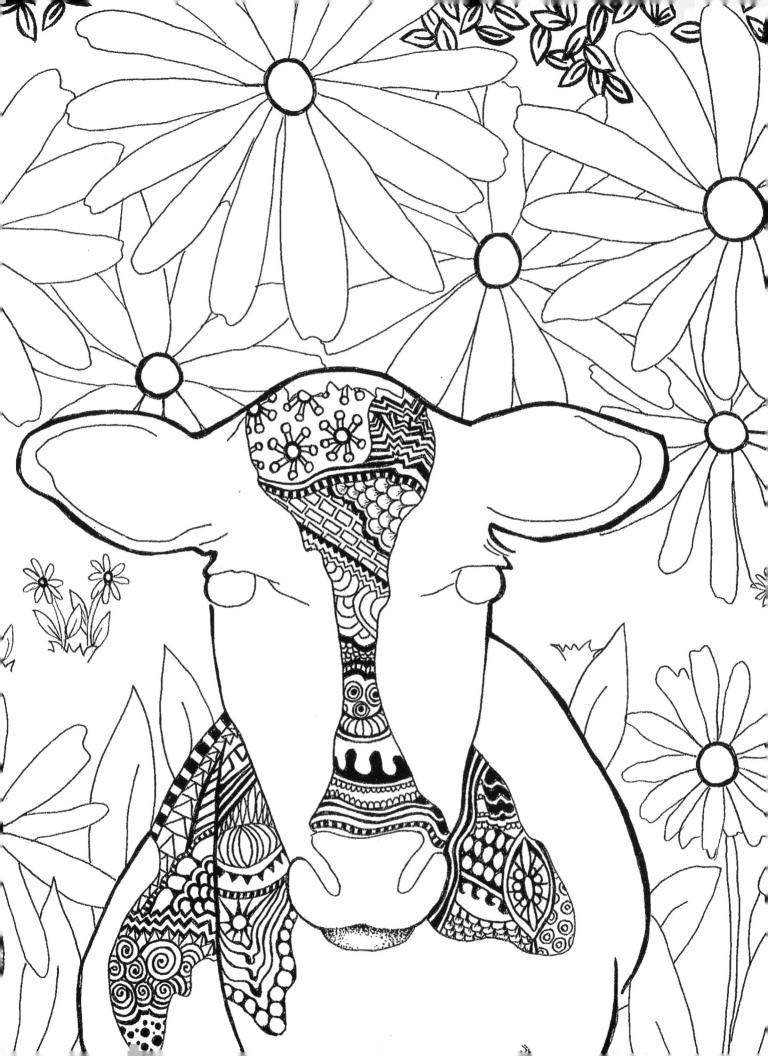

C O W

(BITILASANA)

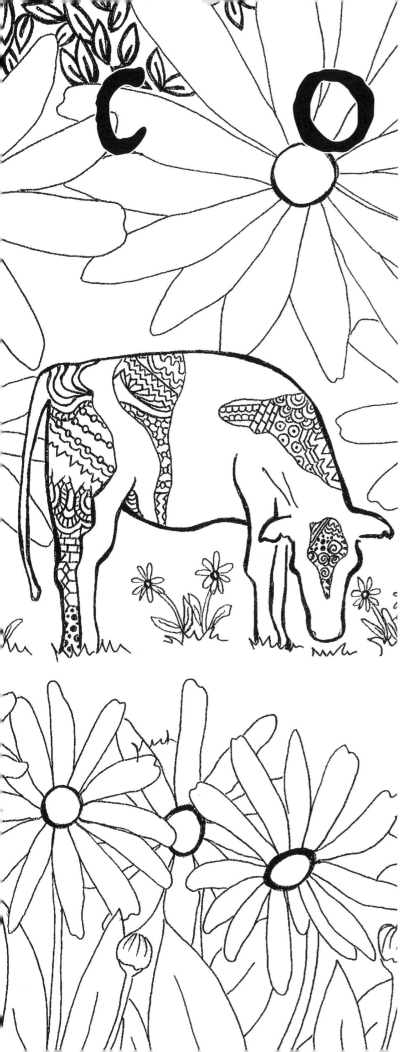

ABOUT THE STRETCH...

Strengthens and stretches the front torso and neck while stretching the hips, abdomen, and back. Massages and stimulates organs in the belly such as kidneys and adrenal glands, while providing a gentle massage.

SETTING IT UP...

From your hands and knees (Tabletop Position) align your hips with your knees to maintain a neutral spine. Press your palms into the ground beneath your shoulders.

As you inhale, lift your sitting bones and chest toward the ceiling, allowing your belly to lower toward the floor. Lift your head to look straight forward.

Cat and Cow pair well together as part of a gentle Vinyasa flow. Start your day with Cat/Cow...you will not regret it!

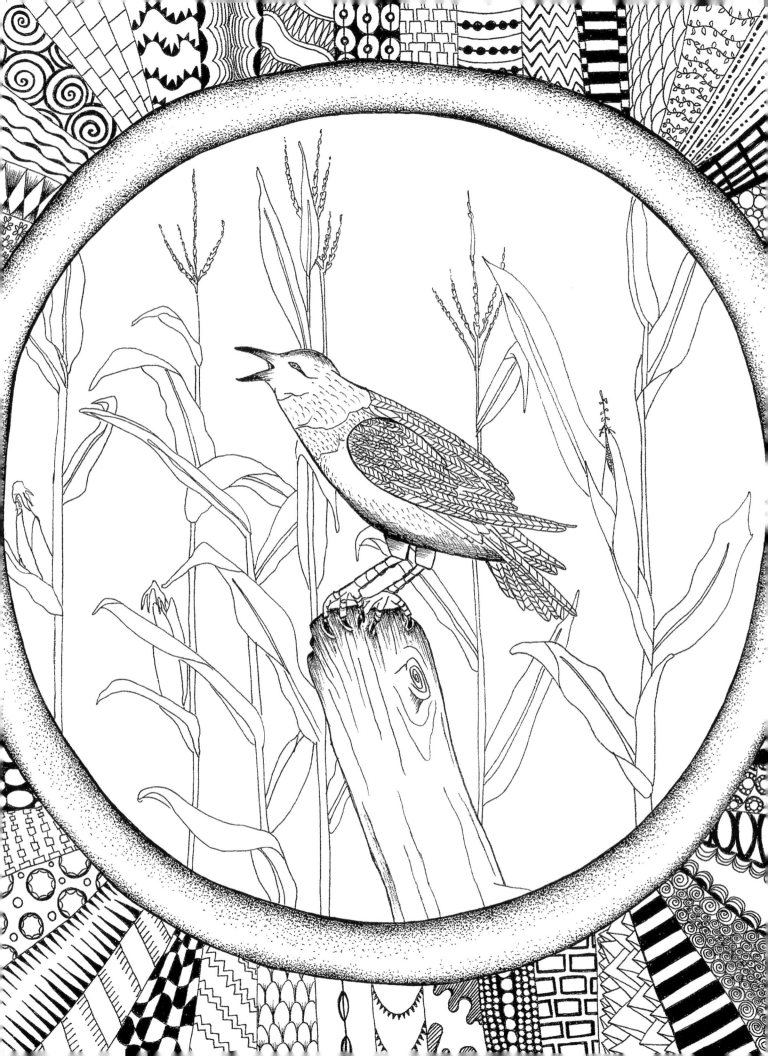

C R O W

(BAKASANA)

ABOUT THE STRETCH...

Strengthens arms, wrists, and core. Stretches the upper back and opens the groin.

SETTING IT UP...

Squat down from Tadasana with your feet a few inches apart. Separate your knees slightly wider than your hips and lean the torso forward, between the inner thighs.

Stretch your arms forward, bend your elbows, plant your hands on the floor. Shimmy the backs of the upper arms against the shins, slowly lifting your feet up off the ground.

Contract your front torso and round your back completely.

Tip: press your feet together and shine your gaze out in front of you.

Tadasana and Malasana set you up to lift up into crow. When your arms start to shake, step or shoot the feet back and flow through your Vinyasa.

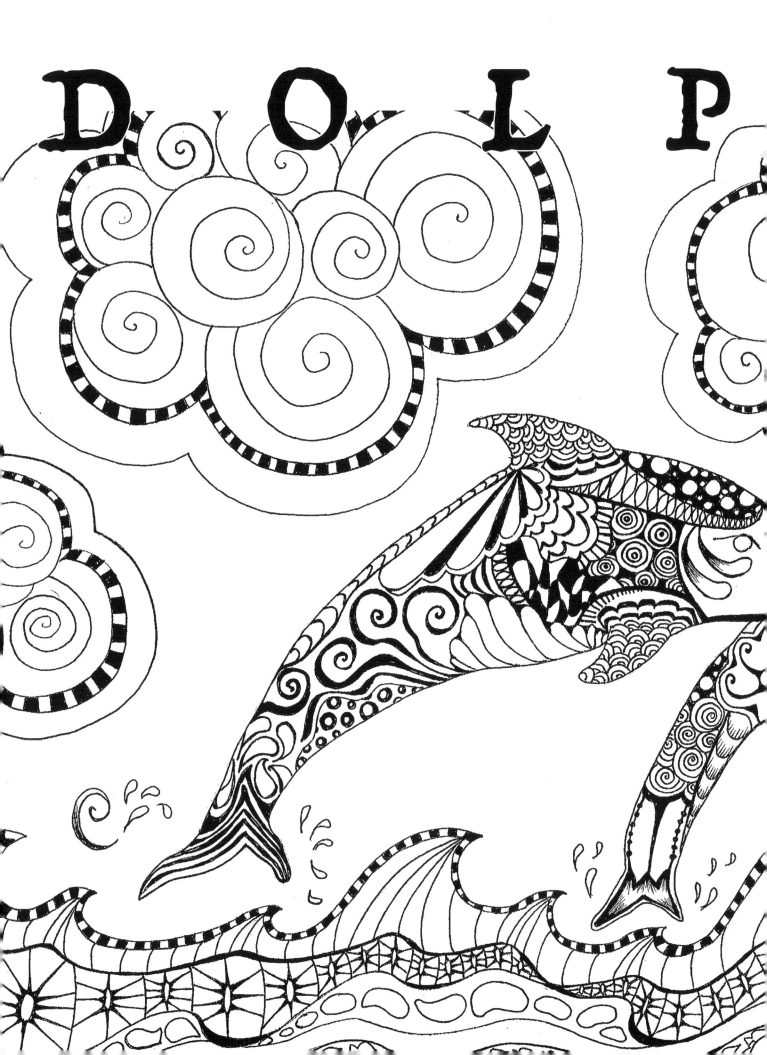

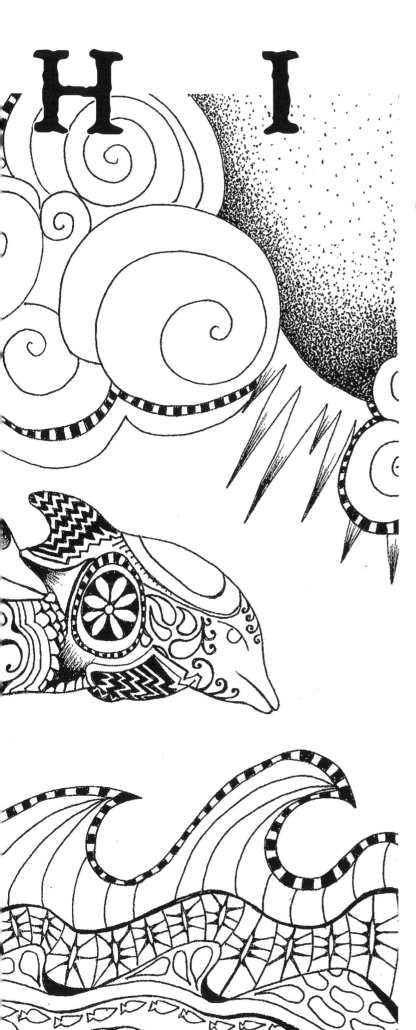

H I N

(ARDHA PINCHA MAYURASANA)

ABOUT THE STRETCH...

Stretches the shoulders, hamstrings, calves, and arches, while strengthening the arms and legs. Calms the brain and helps relieve stress and mild depression. Therapeutic for high blood pressure, asthma, flat feet, and sciatica.

SETTING IT UP...

From your hands and knees, lower forearms to the floor.

Lift sitting bones up while straightening your legs for a modified down dog. Press your heels towards the floor.

Relax your neck and keep space between your ears and shoulders.

Traditional Plank Pose and Forearm Plank are a good warm up before Dolphin. From Dolphin, move into Locust Pose to counter-balance the arms.

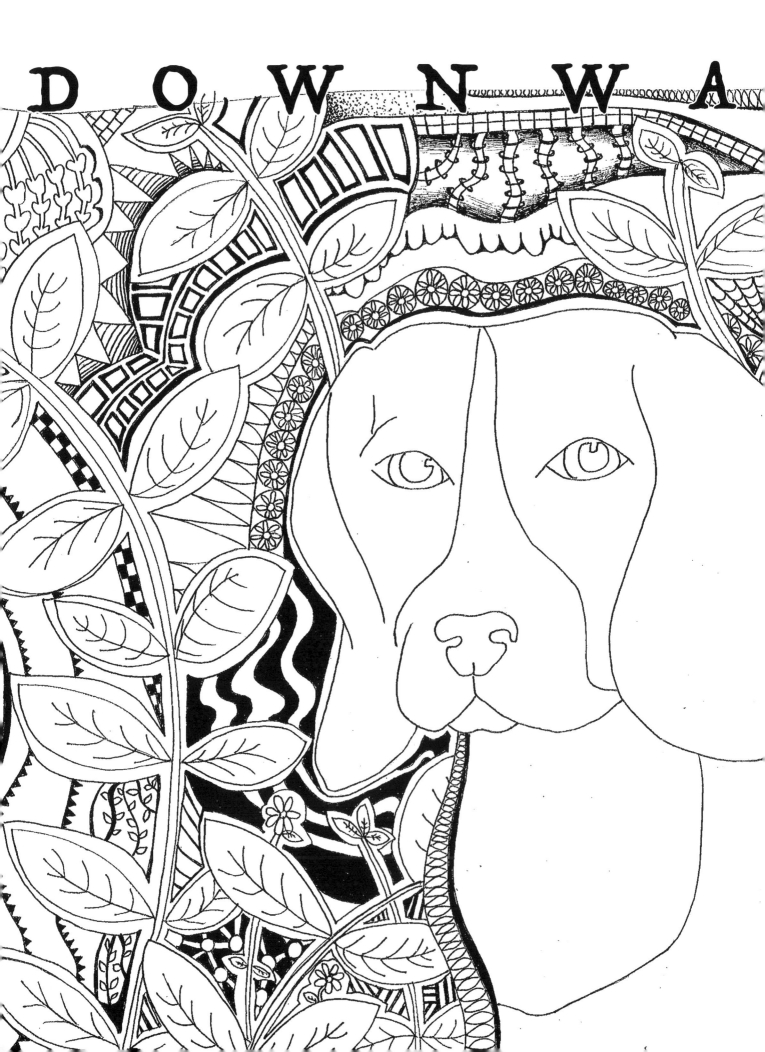

R D D O G

(ADHO MUKHA SVANASANA)

ABOUT THE STRETCH...

One of the most well known yoga poses there is, accessible to babies and elders alike. Calms the brain and helps relieve stress and mild depression, while energizing the body. Stretches the shoulders, hamstrings, calves, arches, and hands while strengthening the arms and legs. Also improves digestion and is therapeutic for high blood pressure, asthma, flat feet, sciatica, and sinusitis.

SETTING IT UP...

From a tabletop position, plant your knees directly below your hips and place your hands slightly in front of your shoulders. Spread your palms, fingers facing forward. Curl your toes under.

Lift your knees away from the floor, creating a triangle shape with your body. Knees can remain slightly bent and heels can be lifted away from the floor. Lift the sitting bones toward the ceiling.

On an exhalation, push your thighs back and stretch your heels onto or down toward the floor. Straighten knees without locking them.

Press the bases of the index fingers actively into the floor. Keep your head between your upper arms; don't let it hang.

This is part of the traditional Sun Salutation sequence and can also be done on its own. To release, lower your knees to the floor.

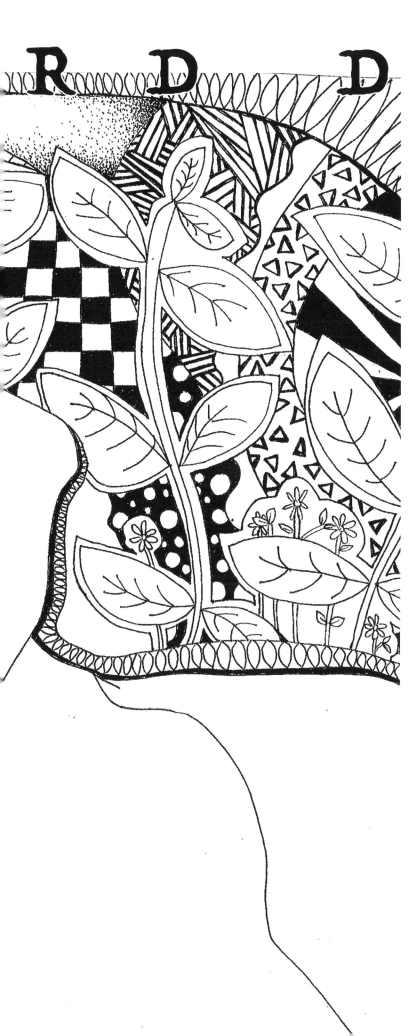

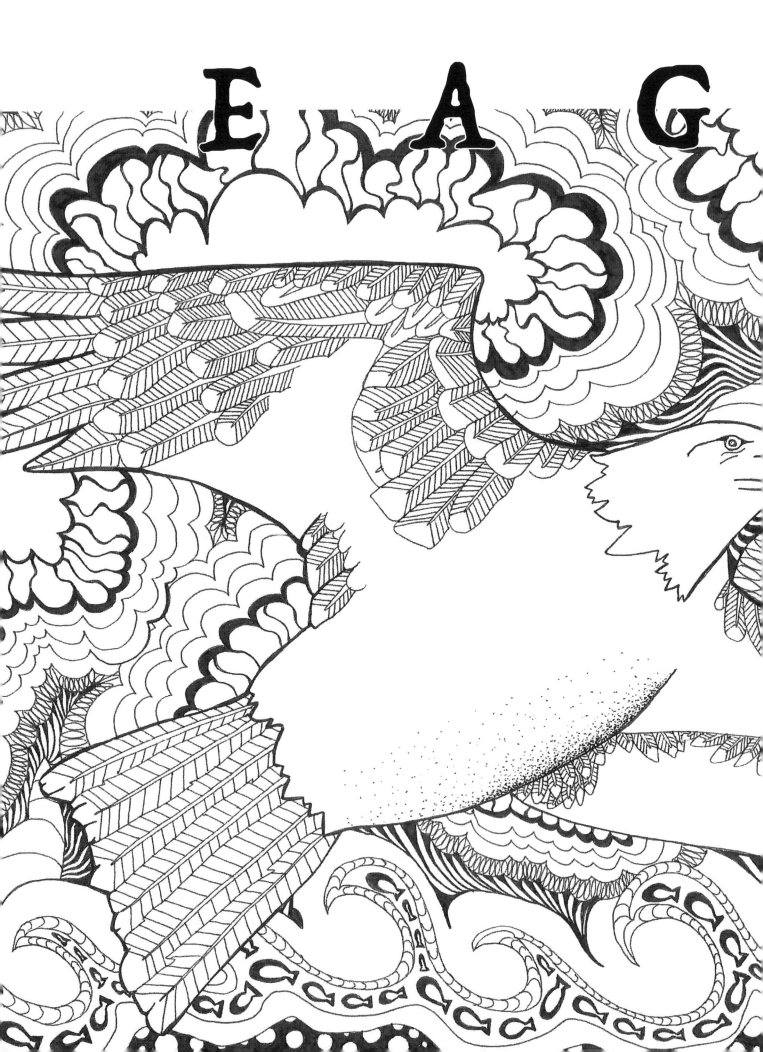

L E

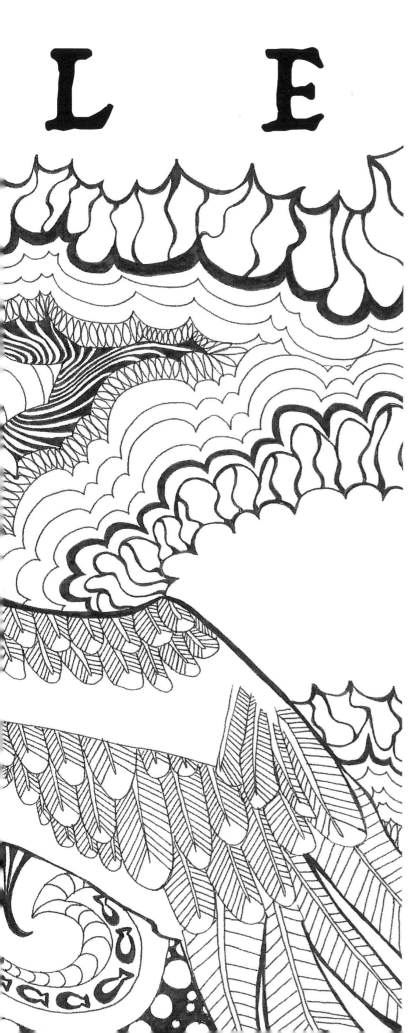

(GARUDASANA)

ABOUT THE STRETCH...

Loosens and strengthens ankles, hips, wrists, and shoulder-full body twister. Releases tightness in shoulders and back while strengthening legs. Cultivates confidence and increases ability to focus.

SETTING IT UP...

From Mountain Pose, cross your right leg over your left (wrap your toes behind your calf if you can.)

Stretch your arms forward before wrapping your right arm underneath your left, pancaking your hands palm to palm.

Sit low into your chair, keeping your gaze on your *drishti* (focal point of view) for balance and focus.

Repeat on second side, crossing your left leg over and wrapping left leg around.

A balance pose, Eagle flows nicely with other standing poses such as Tree, Airplane, and Standing Split.

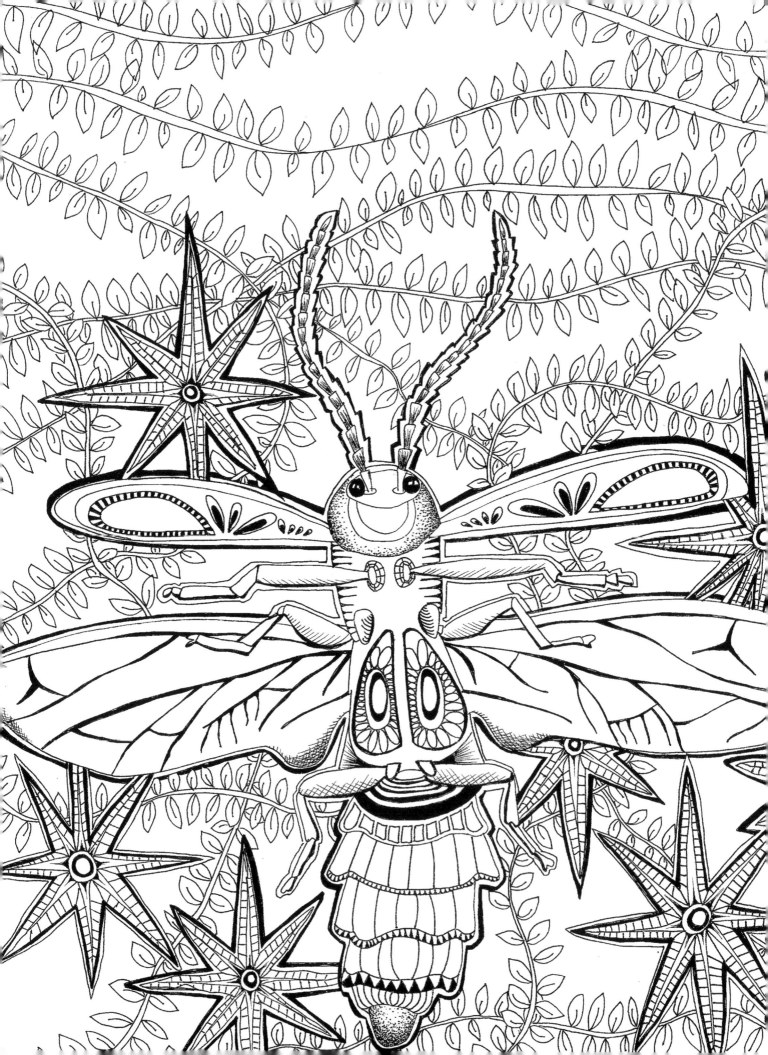

FIREFLY

(TITTIBHASANA)

ABOUT THE STRETCH...

Stretches the inner groin and back torso, and strengthens the arms and wrists. Engages the core to tone the belly. Known to improve sense of balance.

SETTING IT UP...

Squat with your feet shoulder distance apart and bring your trunk between your legs. Straighten your legs enough to lift your pelvis to about knee height.

Bring your left upper arm and shoulder as far as possible underneath the back of your left thigh (just above the knee) and place your left hand on the floor at the outside edge of your foot, fingers pointing forward.

Lift yourself off the floor by pressing your hands into the floor and slowly rocking your weight back. Tip: keep your inner thighs as high on your arms as possible.

With an inhalation, stretch your legs out to the sides as straight as you can, keeping your pelvis high to make your legs parallel to the floor.

Press through the bases of your big toes while pulling your toes back toward your torso. The inner edges of your feet should be angled slightly forward, the outer edges slightly back.

Straighten your arms as much as possible. Hollow your chest as you widen your shoulder blades as much as possible; this will round your upper back, which will lift your torso higher.

This is a challenging pose. You can build up to this by practicing Eagle, Malasana (wide legged squat), Crow and Bound Ankle (Butterfly) poses. Good luck!

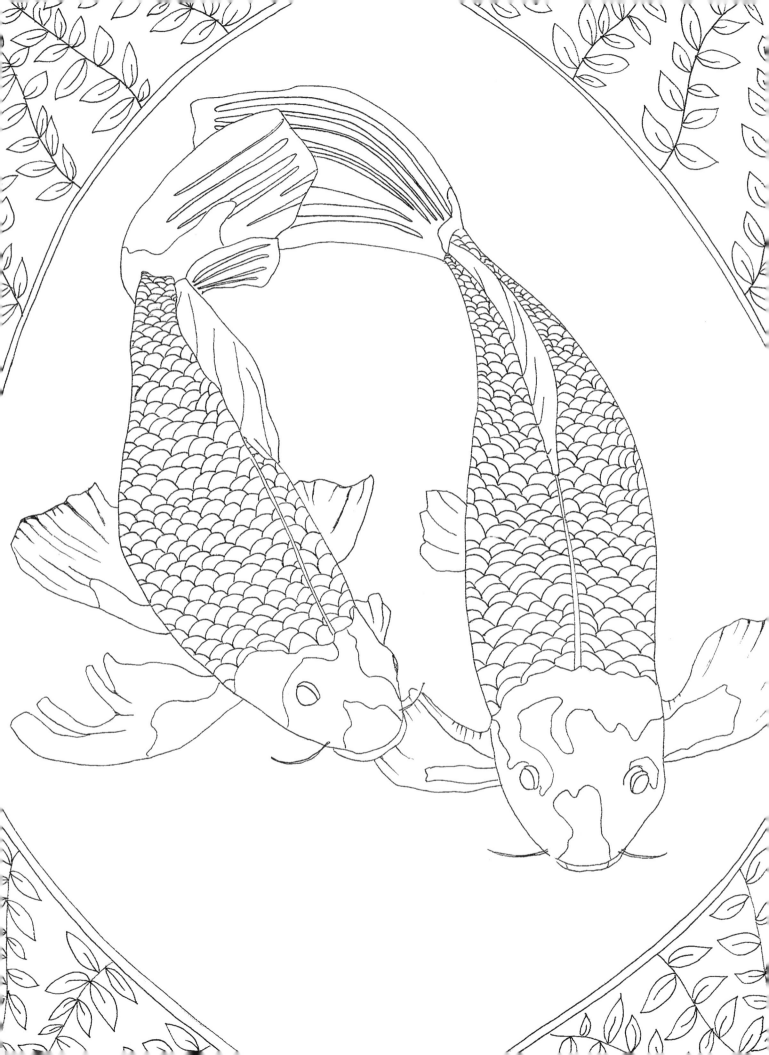

ℱ I S H

(MATSYASANA)

ABOUT THE STRETCH...

Stretches the hip flexors, abdominal and neck muscles, and muscles between the ribs (intercostals), while stimulating the organs of the belly and throat. Also improves posture.

SETTING IT UP...

Lying on your back, inhale, lift your pelvis slightly off the floor, and slide your hands, palms down, below your basement. Rest your basement on the backs of your hands, tucking your forearms and elbows up close to the sides of your torso.

Press your forearms and elbows firmly against the floor, and with an inhale, lift your upper torso and head away from the floor. Release your head back towards the floor with a minimal amount of weight on your head.

Fish Pose often flows with Bridge, Camel, and Hero Pose, which all assist in opening your heart.

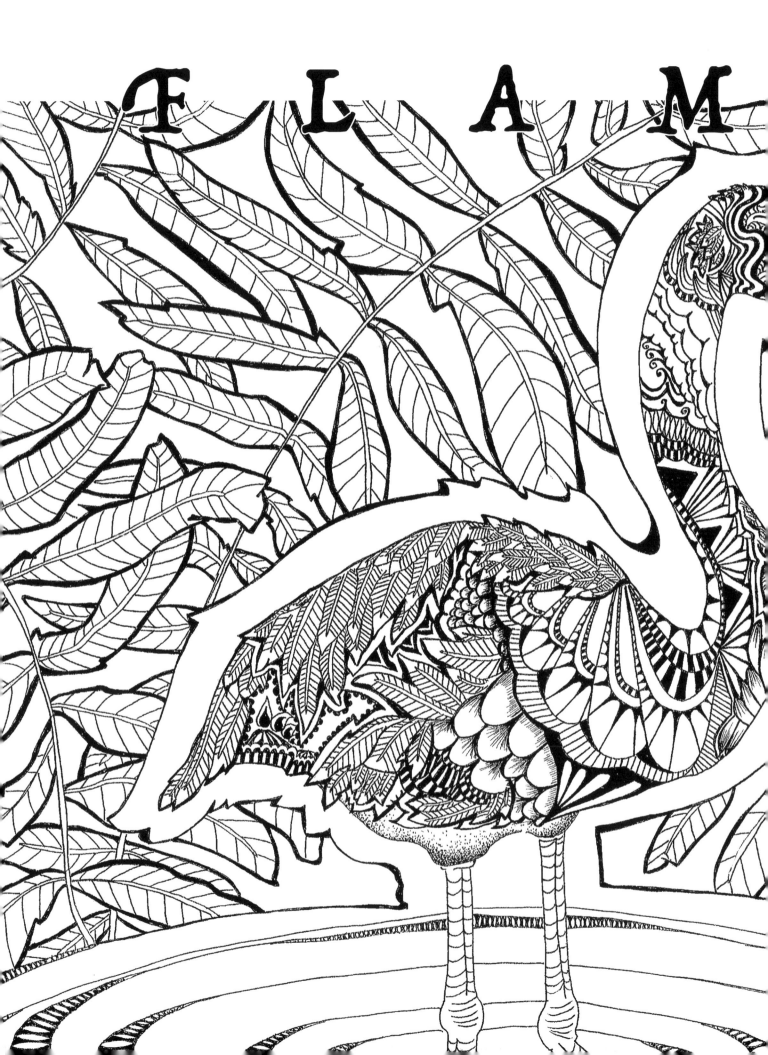

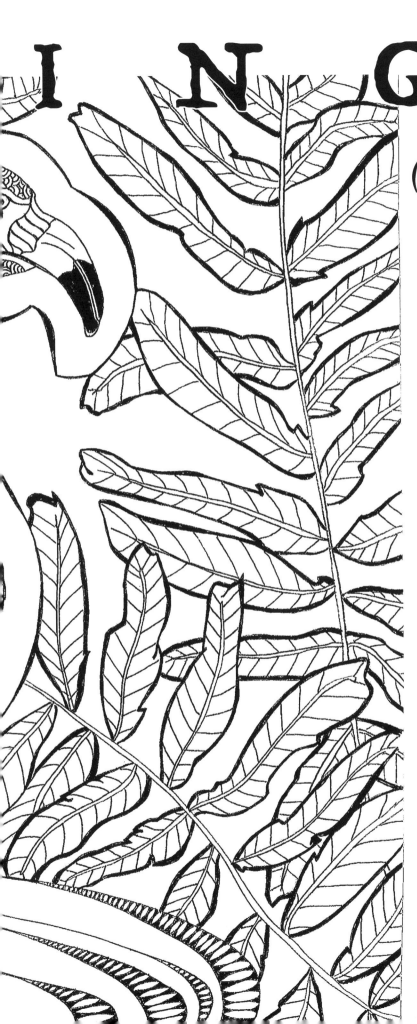

I N G O

(PARSVOTTANASANA)

ABOUT THE STRETCH...

Extreme hamstring opener and forward fold. Strengthens the legs and stretches the spine, shoulders and wrists, hips, and hamstrings. Improves posture and sense of balance. Stimulates the abdominal organs. Invigorating and exhilarating.

SETTING IT UP...

Start with your feet parallel, toes pointing foward and legs wide apart. Interlace your fingers behind your back and hinge foward. Keep the length of your torso directly over your front leg.

Walk your arms back away from your front foot, reaching the fingertips or palms back. Keep your hips square and your spine long.

Pop up onto your fingertip and transfer as much weight into your fingertips as you can.

Deeper? Draw your back heel in toward your bottom for a balance pose.

Parsvottanasana is a good standing pose and prepares you for seated forward bends and twists. Feeling good?

26

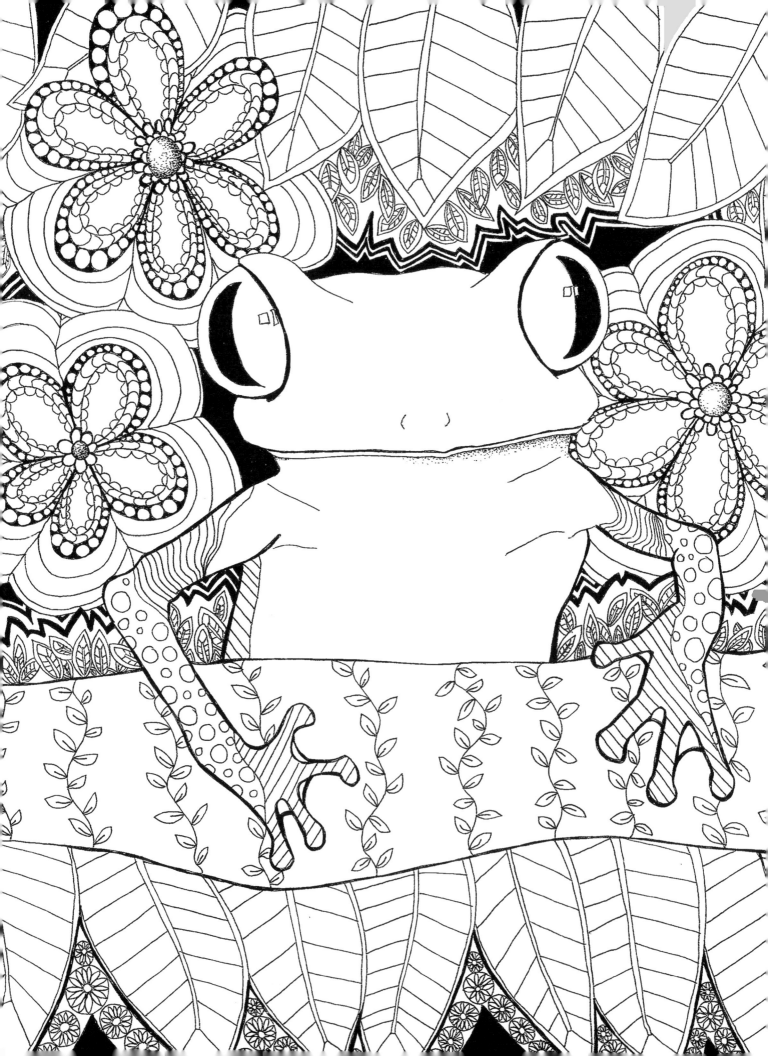

FROG

(ADHO MUKHA MANDUKASANA)

ABOUT THE STRETCH...

Simple and powerful. Opens and stretches hips, groin and insides of the thighs. Releases emotions.

SETTING IT UP...

From your hands and knees (Tabletop Position), walk your knees out to the side as wide as you are comfortable. Keep your ankles directly behind the knees with the feet pointing out.

Bring the elbows, forearms, and flat palms to the floor.

Exhale, press hips towards the back wall, stretch into your hips and inner thighs.

Frog flows best towards the end the end of a practice when your hips and groin are already open. Often followed by a backbend or Shoulder Stand.

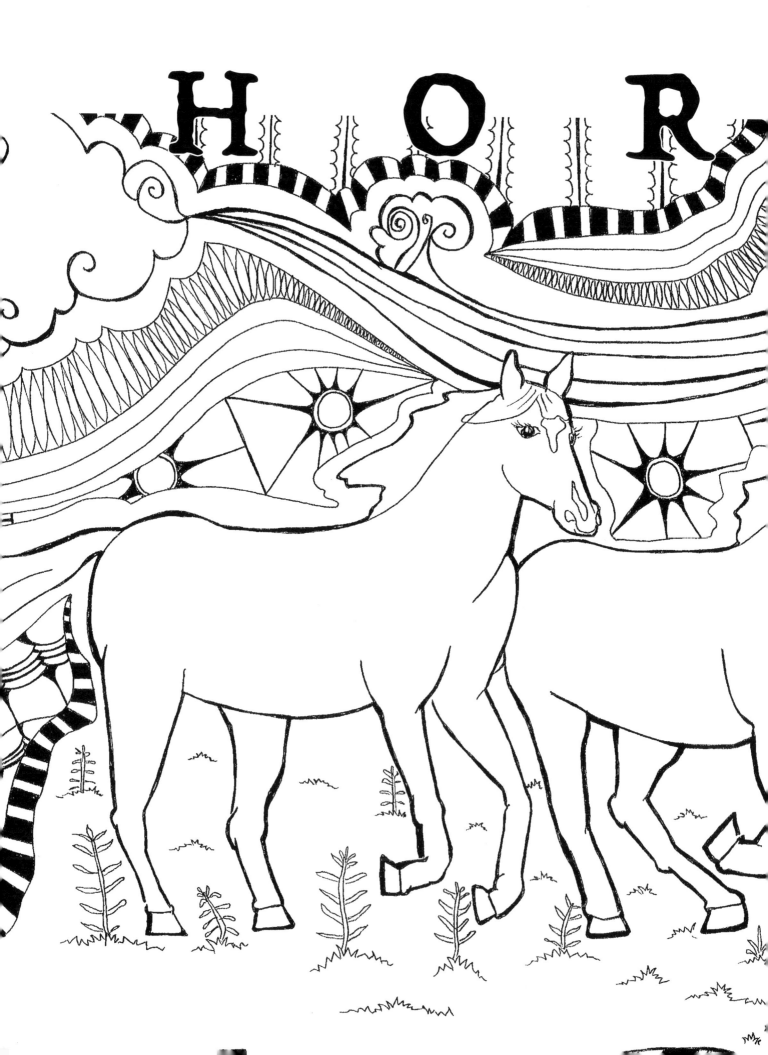

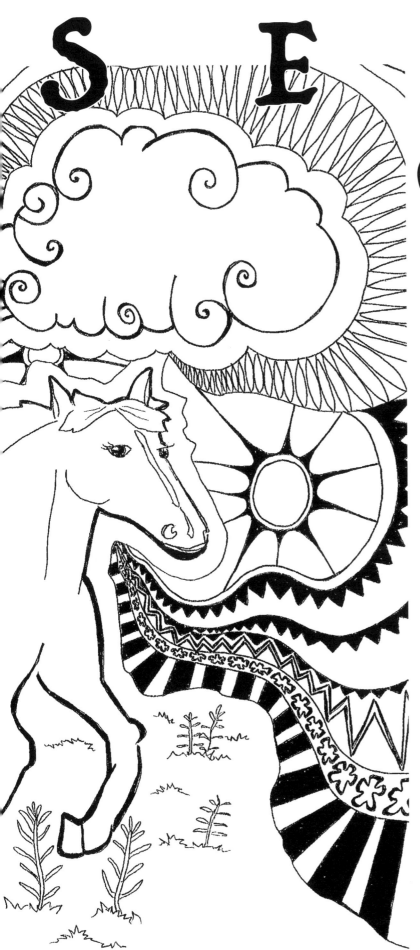

S E

(VATAYANASANA)

ABOUT THE STRETCH...

Creates strength within the legs and openness of the hips, while teaching balance of the body. Focuses on breath and control of the mind.

SETTING IT UP...

With feet slightly turned out, bend both knees and sit your hips down. Make sure your knees are directly over your ankles.

Raise your arms straight up and hold for 30 to 60 seconds.

Horse is a challenging standing pose known to build heat within the body. It sets a strong foundation for the entire practice. Eagle and Lotus offer good preparation for Horse Pose.

30

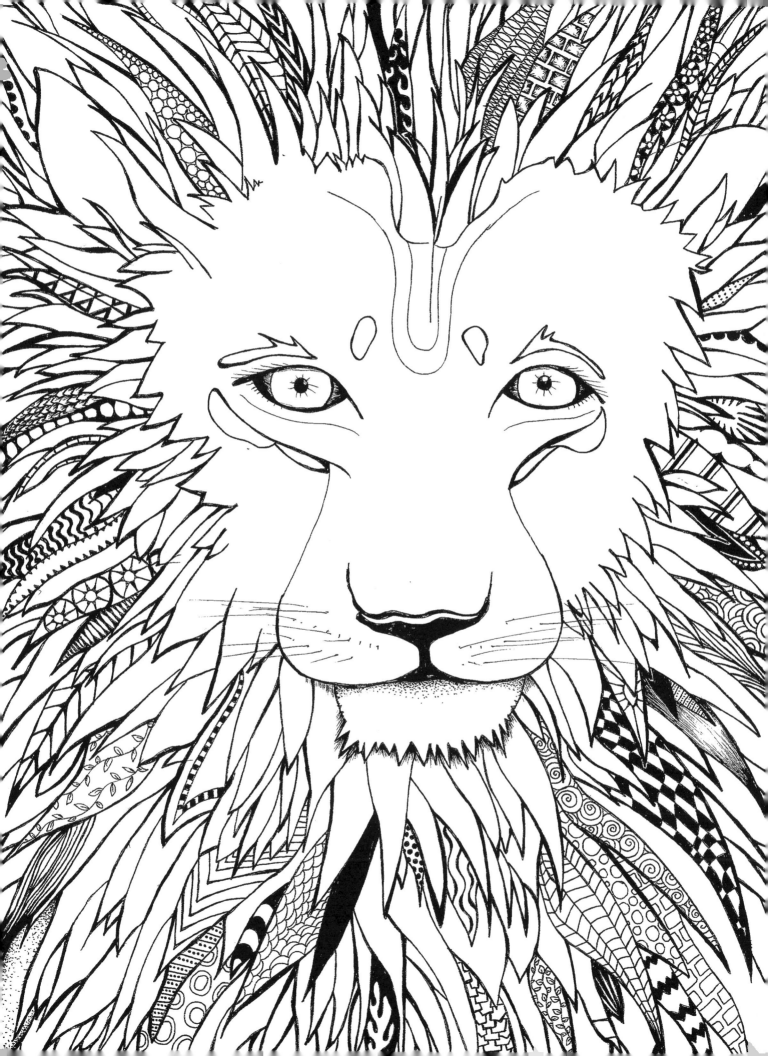

LION'S BREATH

(SIMHASANA)

ABOUT THE STRETCH...

Stretches the muscles in the face, the jaw, and tongue. Relieves tension, tightness, and improves circulation. Energetic and awakening, helping to ease the mind.

SETTING IT UP...

Come to a kneeling position with your basement resting on your feet.

Inhale through your nose and as you exhale through the mouth, make a "ha" sound by opening your mouth wide and sticking your tongue as far out as possible.

Lion's Breath is a warming breath that will increase your internal body temperature and prepare you for any yoga pose.

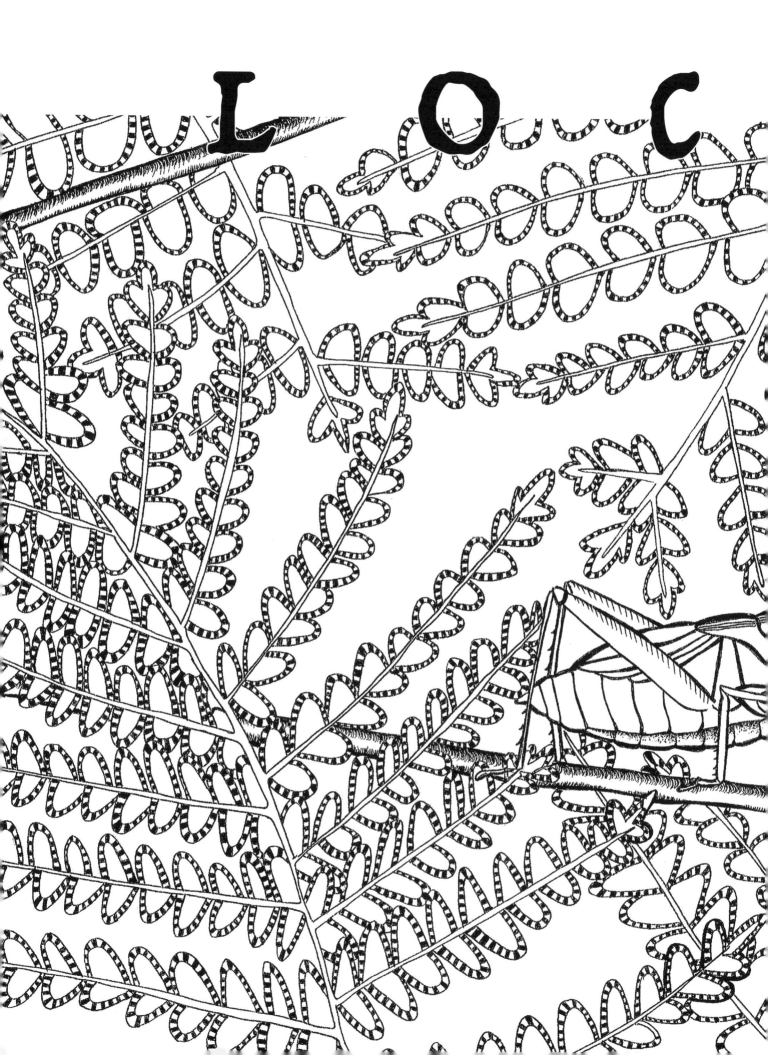

U S T

(SALABHASANA)

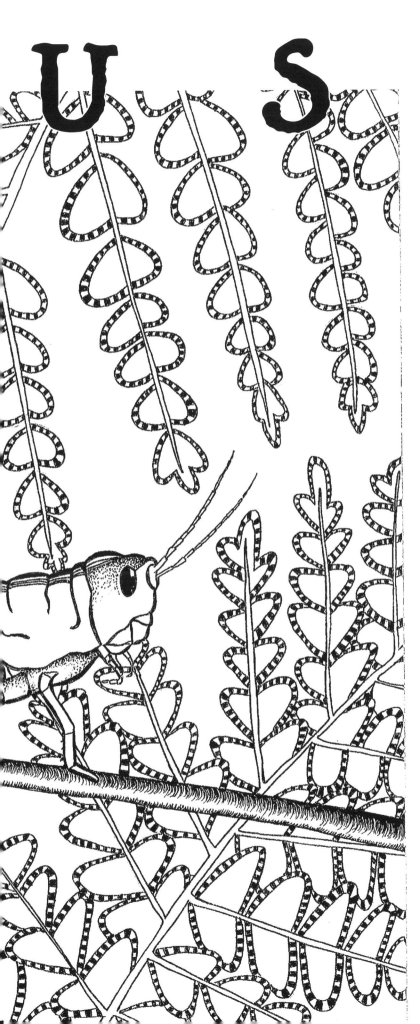

ABOUT THE STRETCH...

Chest opening, back bending, and full body strengthening.

SETTING IT UP...

Lie on your belly with your arms by your sides, palms up, and your forehead resting on the floor.

On an exhale, lift your head, upper torso, arms, and legs away from the floor.

Raise your arms parallel to the floor and stretch back actively through your fingertips.

Cobra, Bridge, and Upward Facing Dog help prepare the back for this. Locust is often followed by twists and inversions.

34

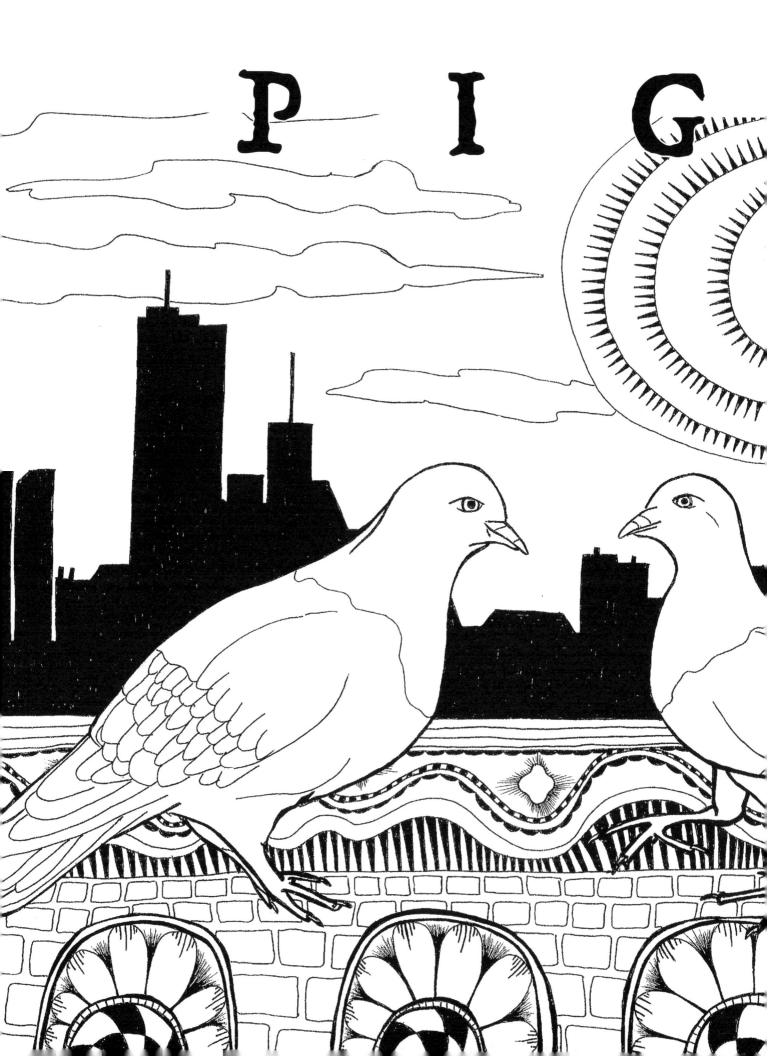

E O N

(RAJAKAPOTASANA)

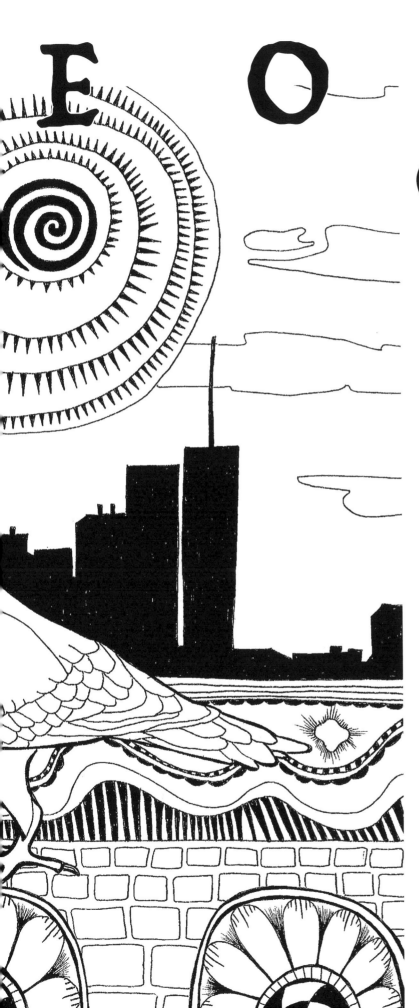

ABOUT THE STRETCH...

Opens up the hip joint and lengthens surrounding muscles while stimulating internal organs. Encourages relief from sciatic and back pain. Releases built up stress, negative energy, and fear.

SETTING IT UP...

From Downward Dog, bring your right knee just behind your right wrist, and place your shin on the floor at a diagonal. Keep your heel pointing toward your hip bone.

With your left leg straight behind you, shimmy your foot back reaching with your toes. Keep that leg in a neutral position and avoid rotating.

Drape your chest over your right leg and release into the mat.

Repeat on second side.

Pigeon is most accessible near the end of a practice when your hips are open. Pigeon leads nicely into Savasana.

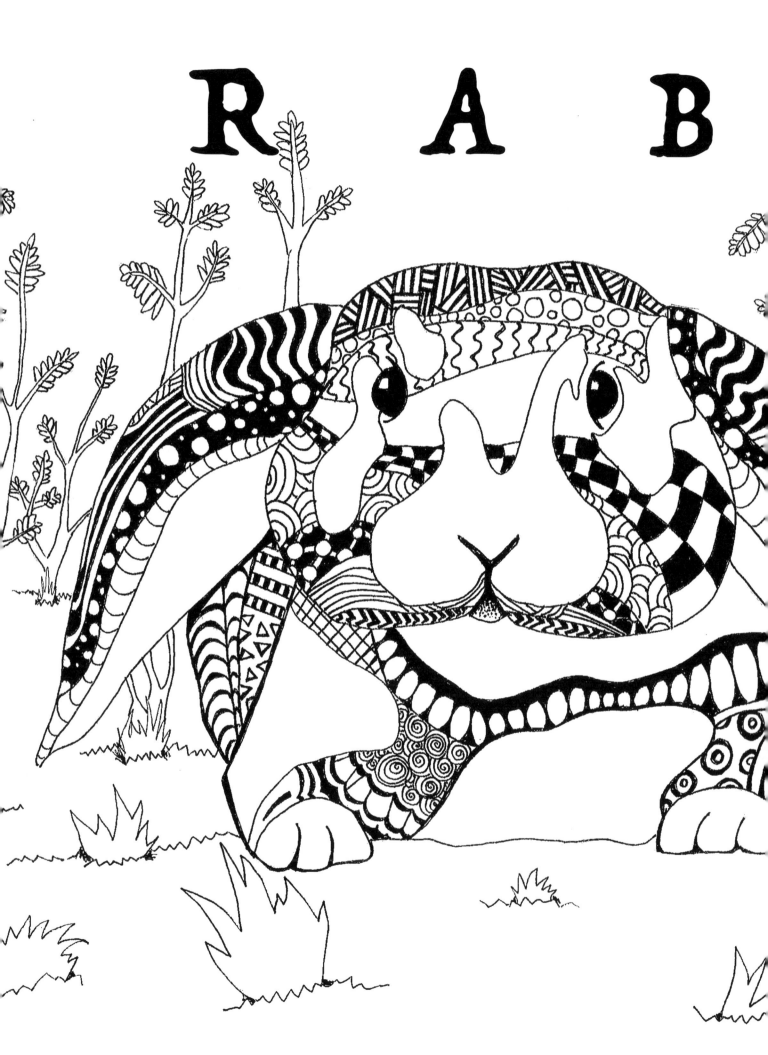

B I T

(SASANGASANA)

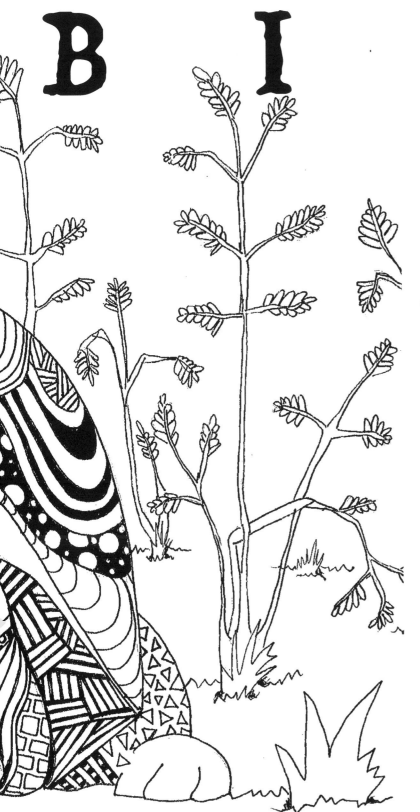

ABOUT THE STRETCH...

Lengthens the spine and stretches the back, arms, and shoulders while stimulating the immune and endocrine systems.

SETTING IT UP...

From Child's Pose, hold onto heels with your hands. Pull your forehead in towards your knees, keeping your forehead on the floor.

Inhale and lift your hips up towards the ceiling, rolling onto the crown of the head.

Press your forehead close to your knees.

Rabbit stretches your back, vertebrae by vertebrae, allowing for alignment and lengthening of the spine. Known to improve posture. Child, Table, Hero, and Camel Poses all lead into Rabbit and can also be transitioned into after coming out of Rabbit Pose.

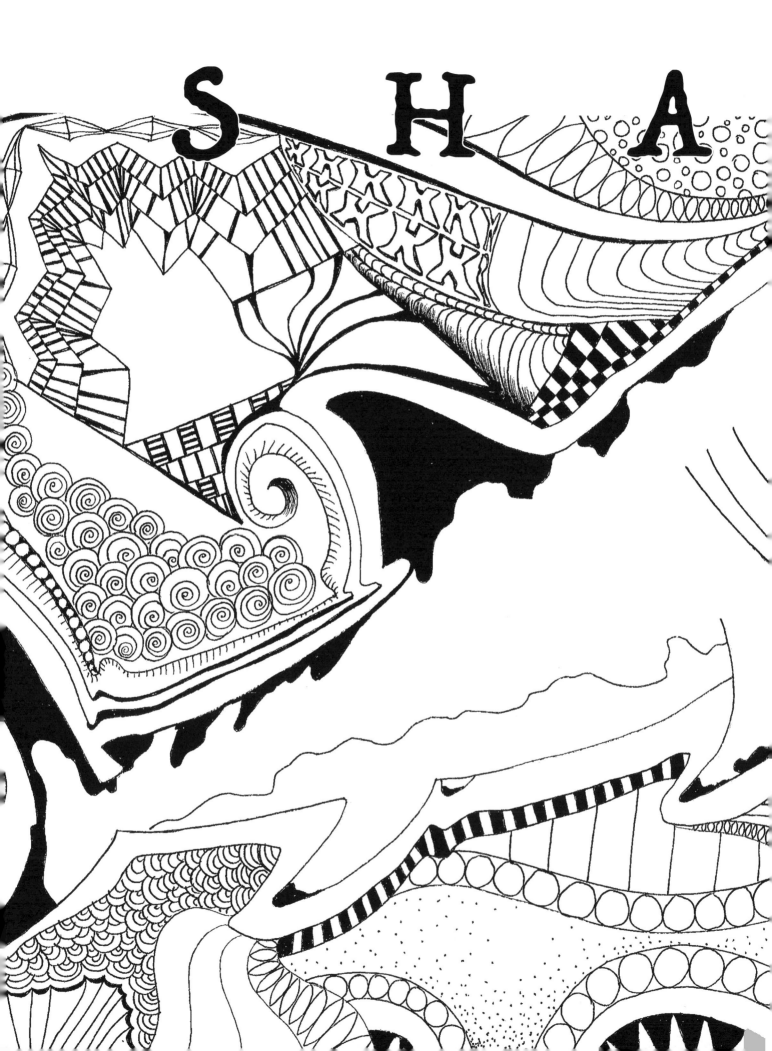

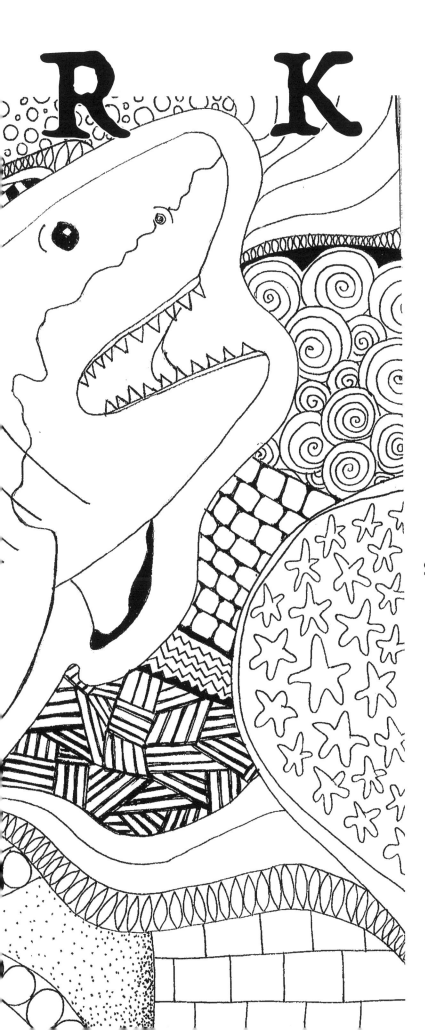

SETTING IT UP...

Flat on your stomach, inhale to lift your legs off the ground, pointing your toes behind you.

Clasp your hands behind your back and lift through the crown of your head.

Feel the massage on your belly and your heart opening up as you hug your shoulder blades into each other. Enjoy the stretch through the crown of your head.

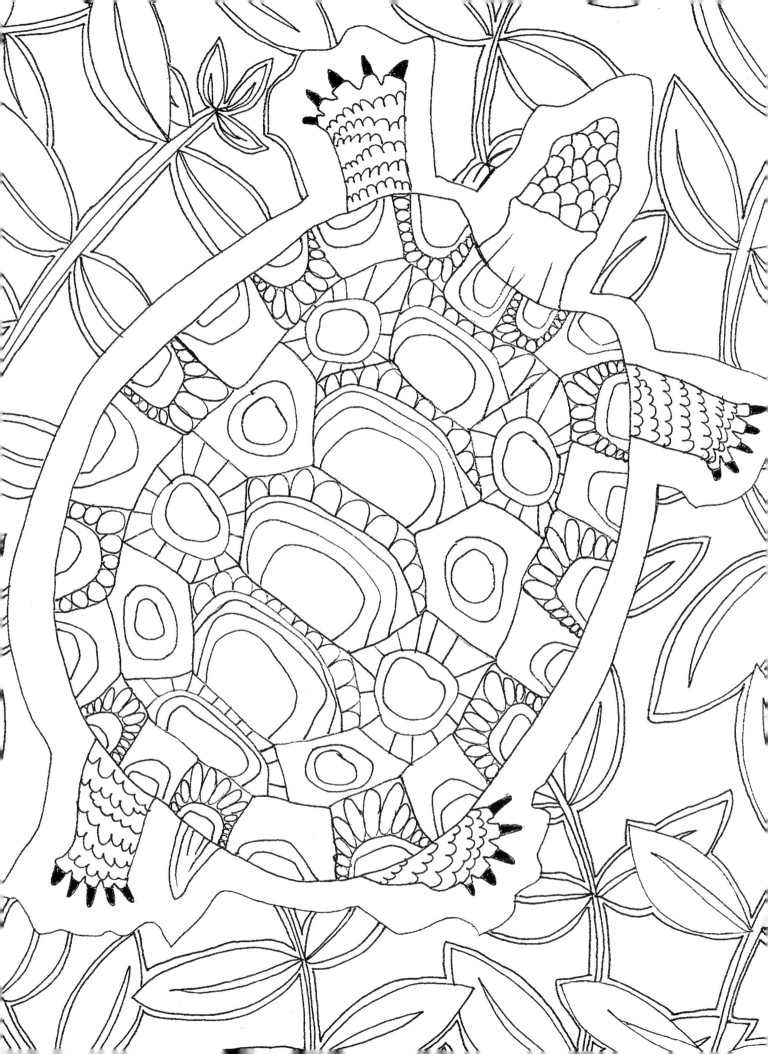

TORTOISE

(KURMASANA)

ABOUT THE STRETCH...

Opens your shoulders and lengthens your spine. Helps you quiet your mind in preparation for meditation. Sounds amazing, right?

SETTING IT UP...

Sit in Dandasana with your legs straight in front of you and your hands on the floor alongside your hips. Bring your legs to the edges of the mat, with your knees as wide as your shoulders.

Bend your knees, and keeping your feet flexed, bring them closer to your hips. Extend your chest and arms forward and down between your legs.

Bend your legs even more so that you can put your shoulders one by one under your knees. (Too hard? Continue to work on forward bends.) Stretching your arms out to the sides, spread the front of your chest and collarbones forward and down. Push your inner heels down and forward. Your inner thighs should remain in contact with your side ribs.

Inhale and exhale to continue extending the spine. (If you are uncomfortable, take your arms slightly forward.)

Poses that help prepare you for Tortoise are Forward Fold, Downward Dog, Chair, Eagle, and Extended Side Angle. Follow up poses include Butterfly, Crow, and Malasana.

GLOSSARY

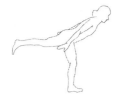 1. AIRPLANE

2. BRIDGE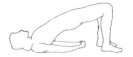

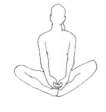 3. BUTTERFLY

4. CAMEL

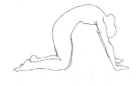 5. CAT

6. CHAIR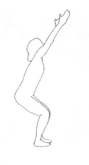

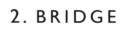 7. COBRA

8. COW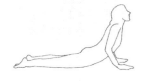

 9. CROW

10. DANDASANA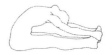

GLOSSARY

11. DOLPHIN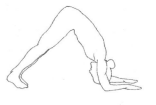

12. DOWNWARD DOG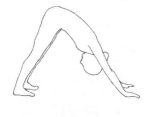

13. EAGLE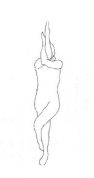

14. EXTENDED SIDE ANGLEGLE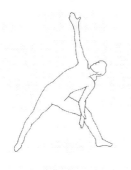

15. FIREFLY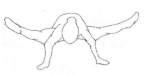

16. FISH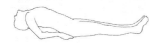

17. FLAMINGO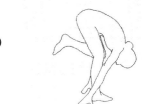

18. FORWARD FOLD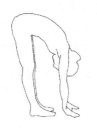

19. FROG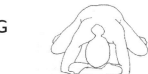

20. FULL WHEEL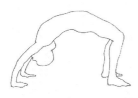

GLOSSARY

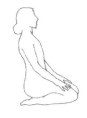

21. HERO

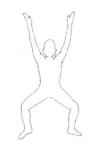

22. HORSE

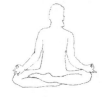

23. LION'S BREATH

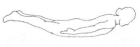

24. LOCUST

25. LOTUS

26. MALASANA

27. MOUNTAIN

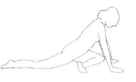

28. PIGEON

29. RABBIT

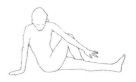

30. SEATED TWIST

GLOSSARY

31. SHARK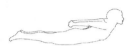

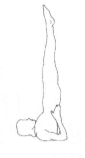 32. SHOULDER
STAND

33. STANDING
SPLIT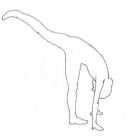

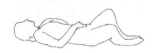 34. SUPTA
PADANGUSTHASANA

35. TABLE TOP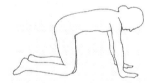

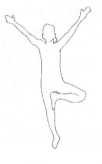 36. TREE

37. TWISTED PUPPY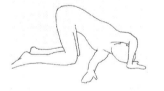

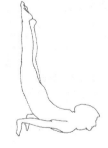 38. UPWARD FACING
DOG

NOTES PAGE

NOTES PAGE

DESIGN YOUR OWN SEQUENCE

DESIGN YOUR OWN SEQUENCE